MR. G. DATESWARAN

C000199914

FIRST AID

Dr D G Delvin

MB BS LRCP MRCS DOBST
RCOG DCH FPA CERT
MRCGP DIP VEN
MFFP

The ROYAL
SOCIETY of
MEDICINE

SUNBURST BOOKS

Editorial Advisor

DR KATHARINE A ORTON
MB BS MRCGP
DCH DRCOG

This edition first published in 1995 by
Sunburst Books, Deacon House,
65 Old Church Street, London SW3 5BS.

ISBN 1 85778 159 7

Printed and bound in China

INTRODUCTION

Welcome to this quick reference guide to first aid; reading it could help you to save someone's life.

Even if you never find yourself in a potential life-saving situation, this book will equip you to deal confidently with the many minor injuries which occur around the home and at work.

I suggest you keep the book somewhere where you can lay your hands on it fast in an emergency, such as with your home or car first aid kit. If you haven't got a first aid kit, this book will tell you how to go about assembling one.

Of course no book can be a substitute for proper first aid training. Being taught face to face by an expert is far better than any kind of 'book learning'. That is why I strongly recommend that you also attend one of the excellent courses run by any of the following first aid organisations:

* In England, Wales and Northern Ireland: St. John Ambulance (London) British Red Cross Society (London)

* In Scotland: St. Andrew's Ambulance Association (Glasgow)

* In the Republic of Ireland: Irish Red Cross Society (Dublin)

* In the USA: American Red Cross (Maryland)

*In Australia: Australian Red Cross
(East Melbourne)

*In New Zealand: NZ Red Cross
(Wellington)

There are also Red Crescent or Red Cross organisations in 146 other countries.

If it simply isn't practicable for you to go on a first aid course, this little book should see you through most of the crises you will encounter – provided you keep your head. Staying calm is the most important principle of good first aid.

Finally, before you use the book, do please read the important warning that follows.

Good luck, and good first aiding.

Dr David Delvin

WARNING

Please read the following very carefully:

* First aid principles vary from country to country. Be guided by the standard practice in your part of the world – there may be a very good reason why something is done in a slightly different way to the one given here.

* First aid practice changes as the years go by – as medical knowledge increases, and the circumstances of life alter. Do not be put off if a bystander tells you that what you are doing isn't what he was taught 30 years ago (this kind of bystander is very common indeed).

* Similarly, bear in mind that some of the principles laid down in this book will eventually be superseded by new ones. Be prepared for this – and be flexible.

* Remember: having this book does not make you a fully trained first aider. In an emergency situation, you must defer to the knowledge of any one with more experience in this field, including not only qualified first aiders, but also doctors and trained nurses.

* If there is anything that you do not understand in this book, you MUST seek expert advice before trying out the technique described.

* If in doubt, it is better to go for what doctors call 'masterly inactivity', rather than doing something which might harm the patient.

ARTIFICIAL RESPIRATION (*see **Mouth-to-Mouth***)

ASPIRIN OVERDOSE
Aspirin overdosage is common, so always stick to the stated dose – and keep aspirin-containing products well out of the reach of children.

Possible symptoms of overdose include:

* Ringing in the ears

* Pain in the upper part of the abdomen (tummy)

* Nausea

* Vomiting (the material may be black or bloodstained)

* Mental confusion

Do not delay. If the person is conscious, get him to hospital immediately. Take any empty tablet bottles with you and also any vomited material – both these items can help the doctors. Do not attempt to make the casualty vomit.

If the person is unconscious, turn to the section on **Unconsciousness** and follow the advice given there.

Do not let anybody destroy suicide notes or unused tablets.

ASTHMA

Asthma attacks are caused by narrowing of the breathing passages. Usually, the victim sits gasping for air and wheezing. She will probably tell you that she has asthma, and may well know how to cope with the attack. It is likely that she will have medication with her.

Your first objective should be to calm her down, then find her somewhere comfortable to sit – preferably well away from crowds of onlookers.

Ask her if she has any medication with her, and whether she should take it. Very often this will be a little aerosol which she puffs into her mouth. Finally, let her rest until she has recovered.

If she does not start recovering rapidly (within 5 minutes), and is obviously in distress, call a doctor or an ambulance. Stay with her until the medical help arrives.

BACK INJURY AND BACK PAIN

If a person has pain in the back but has not injured himself, then there is no real need for first aid intervention. Encourage him to consult his own doctor as soon as possible.

However, if someone has injured his back – say, by falling from a height, diving into shallow water, being involved in a road accident, or being struck a heavy blow, things are very different.

The great danger here is that the spinal cord – the body's main 'nerve cable' – could be damaged. Under these circumstances, sensible first aid can prevent paralysis for life; unwise first aid may cause it. So proceed as follows:

1 Do not let anyone move the casualty.

2 Reassure the casualty, and tell him that he must not attempt to move.

3 Support his head in the position shown in Figure 1. Maintain this support until medical help arrives.

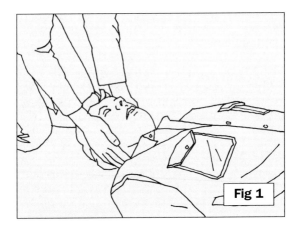

Fig 1

4 Ask someone to call an ambulance.

5 If there are other people around, ask them to get pillows, cushions, coats, etc., and use them to support the casualty's shoulders and neck, as shown in Figure 2.

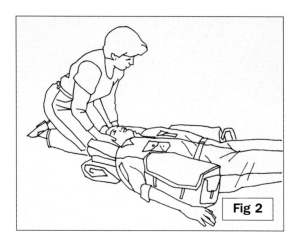

Fig 2

6 If there is traffic nearby, ask someone to direct it safely – so that it does not hit the casualty (or you).

7 If you are far from medical help, and it seems unlikely that an ambulance, doctor or helicopter will reach you within a couple of hours or so, then consider the possibility of getting someone to make a supporting collar for the casualty. You must not let go of the casualty's head until the collar has been fitted, but after that you will have your hands free to tend the victim. However, if you have the slightest doubt about your helper's ability to make a safe collar, then don't ask him to do it. Instead you will just have to keep on supporting the casualty's head with your hands.

8 To make a supporting collar, follow the steps shown in the three illustrations on the next page:

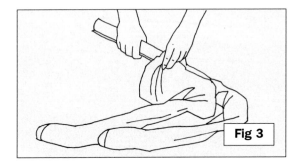

Fig 3

Roll a magazine or thick newspaper into a cylinder – it must be able to bend easily – and wrap it in a piece of cloth. A pair of tights (as shown in Figure 3) will do fine.

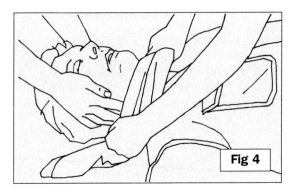

Fig 4

Now you have a collar. Put the centre of the collar directly under the casualty's chin, as shown in Figure 4.

WITHOUT MOVING THE CASUALTY'S HEAD, pass the ends of the collar around the back of his neck and then tie gently at the front (Figure 5).

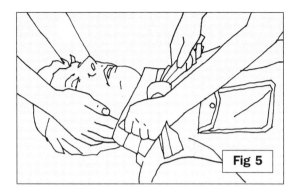

Fig 5

BANDAGES

If you take the advice in the introduction, and go on a first aid course, you will be taught how to apply bandages scientifically and skilfully.

All this short book can do is provide you with some useful tips on different types of bandage and when to use them, and also tell you how to avoid doing harm instead of good when you bandage somebody up.

You can use bandages for four main purposes:

* To stop bleeding

* To support an injured part of the body

* To keep an injured part from moving around

* To prevent an injured part from swelling up

Types of bandage There are various types of bandage, and if you have access to a first aid kit (*see* **First Aid Kit**), it should contain some of each kind. These are the main types:

* Roll bandages, which come rolled up inside a packet – they can·be any thing from 2 cm (0.8 in) to 15 cm (6 in) wide, and are usually at least 1 metre (3 ft) long

* Tubular bandages, which go over the end of a limb, finger or toe

* Triangular bandages, which are used to cover quite large areas, and also to make slings (*see* **Slings**)

Applying tubular bandages requires considerable skill, so we are only going to deal with roll bandages here.

Applying roll bandages Follow these steps:

1 Calm and reassure the casualty.

2 Make sure that the part you are going to bandage is supported – in cases of minor injury, the casualty may be able to do this herself (for example, steadying her injured arm with her good arm).

3 Do not bandage from behind the casualty – do it where she is able to see what you are doing (preferably just to one side of her).

4 Try not to move the injured part any more than you have to.

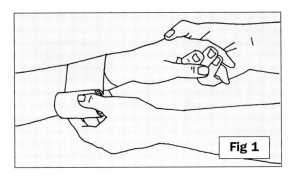

Fig 1

5 Begin by putting the loose end of the bandage on the casualty's skin, then anchor things by making two turns with the roll, as shown in Figure 1. Note from the illustration that while making these two turns, you have the roll of bandage on top (i.e. nearer you).

6 Now make 'spiral' turns with the bandage, so that each turn partly covers the one below, as shown in Figure 2.

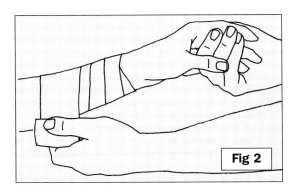

Fig 2

7 Finish by making a couple of 'straight' turns and securing the bandage with a safety-pin, as shown in Figure 3. Take care not to stick the pin in the casualty!

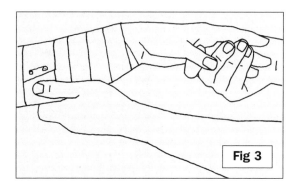

Fig 3

Hand and foot bandaging The type of bandaging described above will get you by in most situations, provided you heed the warnings below. However, it cannot be used to bandage a hand or foot. Instead, use the method shown in Figures 4, 5 and 6.

Figure 4. Make two turns around the ankle or wrist as shown – to anchor the bandage – and then sweep the bandage diagonally across the foot or hand.

Figure 5. Now take the bandage straight under the foot or hand and bring it up the other side.

Figure 6. Bring the bandage diagonally back towards the ankle or wrist as shown, and then finish off with a couple of straight turns and a safety-pin.

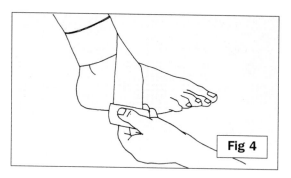

Fig 4

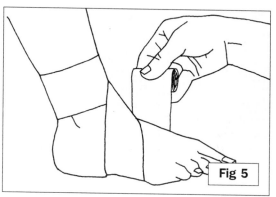

Fig 5

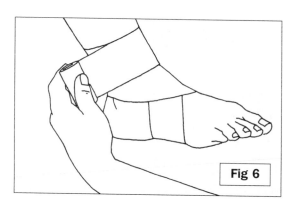

Fig 6

WARNINGS:

* You must not tie a bandage so tight that it stops the circulation of the blood. If in doubt, ease off a bit.

* When bandaging the legs, feet, arms or hands, try to leave the toes or fingertips uncovered if possible.

* If the toes or fingertips go pale, numb or blue, the bandage is too tight, and you must loosen it at once.

* Check the casualty's toes or fingertips every few minutes, until medical help arrives.

* Make sure that your knots do not cut into the casualty.

BITES

If you live in a country where rabies exists (and that means most of the world), always take an animal bite seriously, no matter how minor or insignificant it may look. The casualty MUST go to a doctor for a check-up and a rabies injection.

Quite apart from this, all animal bites are likely to be contaminated by germs, so wash the bitten area very thoroughly with soap and water.

Control any bleeding (see **Bleeding**). Apply a bandage if you have one; if not, cover the bite with a clean cloth. Make sure the casualty goes to a doctor or hospital, because an anti-lockjaw (tetanus) jab will probably be needed.

The same measures are required for human bites, especially as these days there is a small risk of HIV infection.

BLEEDING
Decide at the outset whether the victim's bleeding is trivial or serious. In trivial bleeding, there is little more than a few drops of blood. Anything else should be regarded as serious.

Trivial bleeding. All you need to do is:

* Reassure the casualty

* Clean the wound with soap and water

* Dry the wound

* Cover the wound with a sticking plaster (*see Sticking Plasters*)

* Decide whether it is necessary to take the casualty to a doctor

Don't waste time on trivial bleeding if there is something more important that needs doing – such as ensuring that the casualty can breathe.

Serious bleeding Your prompt action may save a person's life or prevent serious illness. Proceed as described overleaf:

1 You must stop the bleeding – this is best done by really firm, direct pressure on the bleeding point. Press a clean cloth or pad very hard onto the bleeding area, as shown in Figure 1.

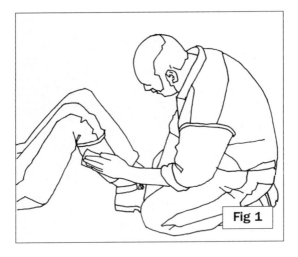

Fig 1

2 Keep up the pressure continuously, for at least 15 minutes (or until medical help arrives). Resist the temptation to 'peek' under the pad.

3 Right from the start, try and raise the part that is bleeding, as shown in Figure 2 – the higher above the heart the better.

4 If something (e.g. an arrow) is sticking out of the wound so that you cannot get a pad directly onto it, then squeeze the edges of the wound together as shown in Figure 3, and press down firmly.

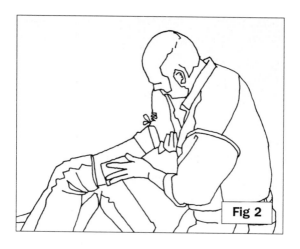

Fig 2

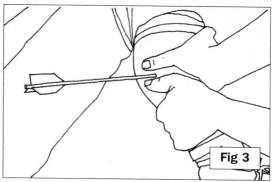

Fig 3

5 Always lie the casualty down – heavy bleeding should never be treated with the casualty in a sitting or standing position.

6 Once the bleeding appears to have stopped, bandage over the wound (see **Bandages**). Do not remove the pad.

7 Stay with the casualty until skilled medical help arrives.

BLISTERS

Do not break blisters. You will do no good, and you may do harm.

Blisters do not need first aid; the best thing you can do is leave them alone.

However, if you think a blister is going to be damaged, for example by shoes, you can cover it with a sterile, non-stick dressing.

BROKEN BONES

Note: A fracture is exactly the same thing as a break.

It is often obvious that a bone is broken – either because someone has heard a 'crack', or because a leg or arm is bent in a funny way.

However, sometimes it is not that obvious. So if you are in any doubt, assume that a bone is broken and treat accordingly until skilled help arrives.

There are two main types of break:

* Those in which the skin is broken (often with a piece of bone sticking out through the skin)

* Those in which the skin is not broken – these are much more common

Breaks in which the skin is not broken

1 Send for medical help.

2 Try to prevent the injured part from being moved by steadying it with your hands, as shown in Figure 1, until someone has found something with which to support it .

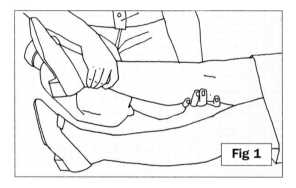

Fig 1

3 For the legs, you will need improvised bandages – scarves, ties or strips of sheet will do. Use them to lash the broken leg gently, but firmly, to the other one, as shown in Figure 2. Or, you can bind the broken leg to something very straight and firm.

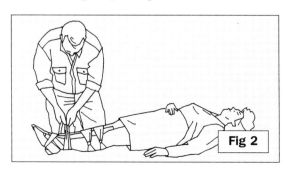

Fig 2

23

4 For the arms, the best thing is to get someone to find some material to make a sling (*see* **Slings**) – a woman's large square scarf is ideal. Or, you can immobilise the injured arm by binding it to something straight and firm, like a walking stick.

Breaks in which the skin is broken These can be much more serious, because there is bleeding, and infection can easily get into the wound.

Proceed as follows:

1 Make sure that somebody has called an ambulance.

2 Steady the injured part, as already described above.

3 Press a clean pad onto the bleeding point, as shown in Figure 3. If nothing else is available, a clean handkerchief will do.

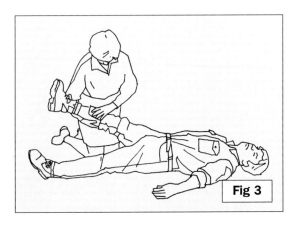

Fig 3

4 If you have some to hand, press cotton wool on top of the pad.

5 If there is a bandage available, wrap it around the pad.

6 Immobilise the limb as described above, and keep it immobile until help arrives.

BRUISES

Minor bruises do not need any first aid.

A big bruise which starts developing very soon after an injury can be 'limited' by prompt first aid.

Proceed as follows:

1 Apply ice to the bruise, but only through a thick cloth, so you do not 'burn' the skin. Keep the ice on for 5 minutes. If you have no ice, a pack of frozen food (e.g. peas) will do.

2 While applying the ice, keep the injured part raised.

3. Apply a bandage to the injured part (*see* **Bandages**) to try and stop it from swelling up. If possible, put a pad of lint or cotton wool on first.

BURNS AND SCALDS

Burns and scalds can both be treated in the same way. (However, for burns caused by chemicals, *see* **Chemical Burns**.)

Remember: the vital thing is to cool the injured part as quickly as possible. If you do not do this, heat damage may continue for some minutes.

Serious burns (if in doubt, treat as serious)
Proceed as follows:

1 Get the victim lying down straight away.

2 Drench the burned part with lots and lots of cold water – the quicker you can start doing this, the better (see Figure 1).

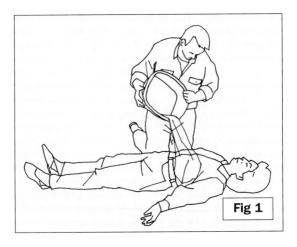

Fig 1

3 Remove belts, watches, bangles or anything else which might cause constriction near the burned area.

4 Remove any smouldering clothing, because it may still be burning the victim.

People who did some first aid a long time ago may try to stop you doing this, but it is now official advice.

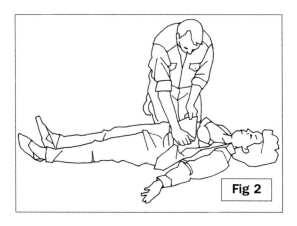

Fig 2

5 Cover the injury with a sterile dressing, or failing that, a freshly laundered, non-fluffy cloth or handkerchief, as shown in Figure 2. Clingfilm or a clean plastic bag can also be used.

6 Do not under any circumstances put any cream or other application on the burn, no matter how 'good' or 'soothing' anybody tells you it is.

7 Make sure that an ambulance has been called. While waiting for it keep the casualty as calm and as comfortable as possible Do not let anyone give him hot drinks or tablets or indeed anything by mouth.

Trivial burns
Proceed as described overleaf:

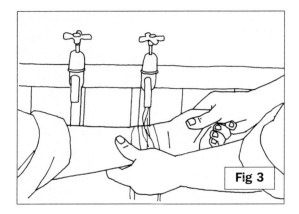

Fig 3

1 Cool the injured part under a running tap, as shown in Figure 3.

2 Cover the burn with a sterile dressing, and put a bandage round it, as shown in Figure 4. Do not tie the bandage tightly. If you haven't got a sterile dressing and bandage, you can use any freshly laundered, non-fluffy cloth.

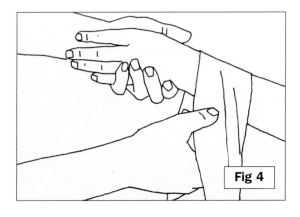

Fig 4

3 Do not apply any cream, ointment, etc. to the burn or scald. And do not put cold tea on it either.

CARDIAC MASSAGE (see *Heart Massage*)

CHEMICAL BURNS

Many chemicals, including acids and alkalis, can cause terrible burns to the skin (and, more particularly, to areas such as the eyes and mouth).

Your prompt action can prevent serious injury. Proceed as follows:

1 Drench the burned area with water, as shown in Figure 1. The longer you do this, the better; if the chemical is a sticky one, you may need to continue drenching the area for up to 15 minutes. Do not let yourself be hurried by well-meaning people; take your time.

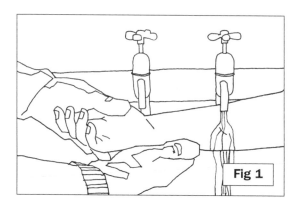

Fig 1

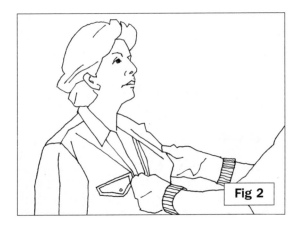

Fig 2

2 If the victim's clothes are soaked in the chemical it will continue to burn her. Gently remove the wet clothes (Figure 2) – wearing rubber gloves if possible – and put them in a safe place where they won't burn anyone.

3 If the chemical has got in the victim's eye, put her head under a running cold tap, as shown in Figure 3. Make sure the water drains away from the eye, not over her face.

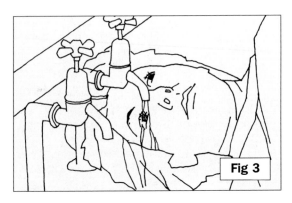

Fig 3

In all cases, make sure that you do not wash the chemical over yourself or other people.

CHILDBIRTH (EMERGENCY)
It is actually quite rare for a first aider to have to deliver a child, because in practice most women in labour do manage to get to a hospital in time.

If you do find yourself faced with an emergency childbirth situation, the most important thing to remember is this. **If you simply reassure the mother and do nothing physical to interfere with the birth process, the odds are heavily in favour of everything turning out OK**. But if you start doing any pushing, pulling or cutting, you could do very serious harm.

Preparation In the unlikely event that you have some minutes or even hours to prepare for the delivery (this can be the case in remote places), then get things ready as follows:

1 Prepare a comfortable, secluded place for the mother. A room with a bed in it is ideal, and there should be plenty of pillows, so that she can sit up with lots of support behind her back.

2 Get something ready to put the baby in. If there is no cot or pram, a deep drawer from a chest-of-drawers will do fine. Put blankets or some other warm wrapping inside it – remember, if you are in a temperate country, cold is a major threat to a baby's life.

3 Cover the bed and floor with clean towels or, if there are none available, clean newspapers – there will inevitably be some mess when the child is born.

4 Find some clean sheeting or towelling to put under the woman's bottom.

5 Ask everybody to leave the room, apart from those people the mother wants to be present. In particular, keep out anybody who has got a sore throat, cold or any other type of infection.

6 Just as they do in the films, ensure that there is a plentiful supply of hot water for washing things. If there is no hot water supply, get somebody to boil some water.

7 When the birth seems to be getting quite near, wash and scrub your hands very thoroughly in hot, soapy water for a good 5 minutes.

The birth It is far more likely that you will come across a situation (maybe in a street, shop or taxi) where a woman is actually on the brink of producing her baby.

In such a case, proceed as follows:

1 Make sure that someone has rung for an ambulance, and ask someone to get you some clean plastic gloves from a pharmacy.

2 Clear all bystanders – though there may be somebody the mother wants to stay around and hold her hand.

3 Make the mother as comfortable as you possibly can, in as secluded a spot as possible. Put a clean cloth under her bottom.

4 Reassure her that everything will be OK.

5 Help her to lie on her back, with her shoulders comfortably propped up.

6 Ask her to part her legs and to put her hands on her knees, as shown in Figure 1.

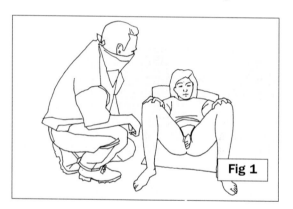

Fig 1

7 Every time she has a pain (contraction), encourage her to push downwards. Tell her not to push between pains.

8 Do not get any crazy ideas about 'holding the baby back' or delaying the delivery. This is impossible.

9 Tie a clean handkerchief over your mouth and nose, to reduce the chance of giving the mother an infection, and put on the plastic gloves if available.

10 Ask the mother's permission to examine her vaginal area. If you can see the baby's scalp, the birth is imminent. If you cannot, then you have plenty of time – and it is probable that the emergency services will be there to relieve you before the baby arrives.

11 Continue to reassure the woman, and to encourage her to push down with the pains (not in between).

12 There will come a moment when the widest part of the baby's head pops out – as shown in Figure 2. At that point, you must tell the mother to stop pushing, and to pant (like a dog) until the whole of the baby has been delivered.

13 Support the baby's head with your hands, as shown in Figure 2. **Whatever you do, do not pull on the baby or try to tug it out.**

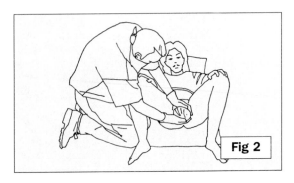

Fig 2

14 If there is a 'film' over the baby's face, brush it away.

15 The baby's face will usually emerge pointing towards his mother's bottom. You will then find that his face turns naturally to the side, as in Figure 3. Do not interfere with this movement – just support the head.

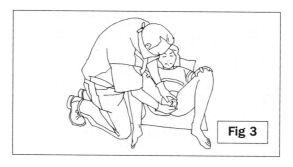

Fig 3

16 You will now be able see the baby's neck. If the cord is wrapped around the neck, gently ease it over baby's head with your finger.

17 The baby's shoulders will now come out. You can help the first shoulder to emerge by lowering the baby's head slightly. The second will emerge more easily if you raise the head slightly, as shown in Figure 4.

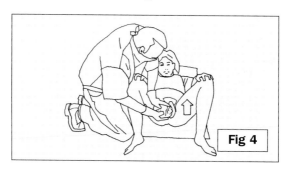

Fig 4

18 The rest of the baby will follow quickly. He will probably be slippery, so be careful not to drop him. Just ease him upwards onto his mother's tummy.

19 The cord runs from the baby's navel back into his mother's vagina. **It is vital that you do not do anything to it**. Do not pull on it, and do not let anyone cut it. It must be left uncut until a qualified person gets there.

20 If the baby is not yet crying, clear his mouth with a clean handkerchief. Do not smack him – it is a myth that this does any good. If he is not breathing within 60 seconds, give him gentle artificial respiration as described in the section **Mouth-to-Mouth** (Treating babies).

21 Once he is breathing, wrap him in something warm, and give him to his Mum to hold.

22 The 'afterbirth' (placenta) will eventually be delivered – it is on the other end of the cord. Do not do anything to this except wrap it up, e.g. in a plastic bag.

23 Put a clean towel or a sanitary pad over the mother's vagina and keep her reassured and comfortable until help arrives.

CHOKING
People frequently choke on something they have 'half swallowed'. This is particularly common in young children, who instinctively put things in their mouths.

What happens is that the object gets jammed at the top of the main air tube (roughly behind the Adam's apple), so that no air can get in or out.

If the obstruction is not removed, the person will die within a few minutes. You can save the victim's life if you act promptly. What you do depends on whether the victim is an adult, a child or a baby.

Adults When an adult is choking, he may stagger around pointing to his throat, but because the air tube is blocked, he cannot tell you he is choking.

Proceed as follows:

1 Bend the victim right forward and, as shown in Figure 1, slap him five times between the shoulder-blades with the flat of your hand.

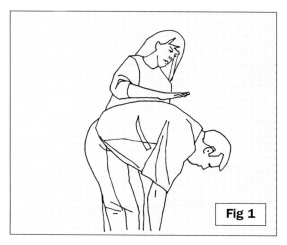

Fig 1

2 If this does not work, you must try Heimlich's technique immediately. Stand the victim up, and place yourself behind him, as shown in Figure 2.

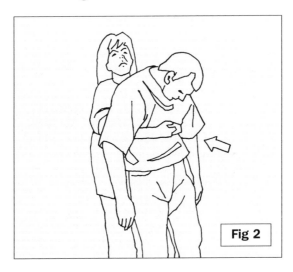

Fig 2

3 Interlock your fingers firmly, as shown in Figure 3, over the upper part of his tummy. Your hands should be several inches above the navel. (If the casualty is a woman, your hands should be well below her breasts.)

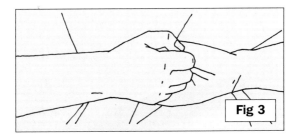

Fig 3

4 With a sudden movement, pull your linked hands very, very hard towards you. Use as much force as you can, in an attempt to drive the breath out of his chest and so 'blast' the obstruction out, like a cork from a bottle.

5 Repeat this movement until you push the obstruction out and the casualty starts to breathe.

6 If you are not successful, the casualty will eventually become unconscious as a result of lack of air. If that happens, put him flat on his back, as shown in Figure 4. Kneel astride him, and put your two hands on the upper part of his tummy as shown.

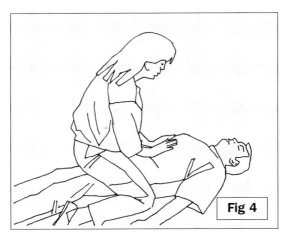

Fig 4

7 Now thrust forcibly in an attempt to drive the air hard out of his lungs. Imagine that you are driving at a point on his back, midway between his shoulder-blades.

8 Repeat these thrusts until you successfully push the obstruction out and the patient starts breathing.

9 Put him into the recovery position (*see* **Unconsciousness**), and stay with him until help arrives.

Children If a child under the age of 10 is choking, it is best not to use the Heimlich technique. Instead, proceed as follows:

1 Sit on a firm chair, and put the child over your knee, face down. If you are right-handed, have his head on your left.

2 Make sure that his head is well below the level of your knees, as shown in Figure 5.

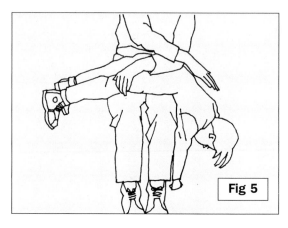

Fig 5

3 Slap him repeatedly between the shoulder-blades with your open right hand, as shown.

Babies The technique for treating a choking
baby is very similar to that for a child.
Proceed as follows:

1 Sit on a firm chair.

2 Put the child across your lap.

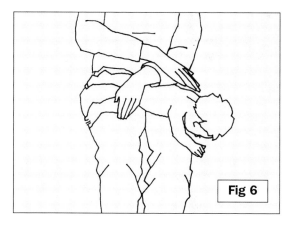

Fig 6

3 Steady him with your left hand on his
hips, as shown in Figure 6.

4 Lower his head, using the support of your
fingers to keep him from falling.

5 With your other hand, slap him gently
between the shoulder-blades.

COLD (EXTREME)
Extreme cold can kill people, and is a
common cause of death in winter, even in
temperate countries. Those most at risk are:

* Old people

* Very young children

* The physically exhausted or injured,
  e.g hill walkers or mountaineers

The word 'hypothermia' just means 'lack of
warmth'. In general, a person is said to be
suffering from hypothermia if her
temperature falls to 35°C (95°F) or below.

The features of hypothermia are:

* Feeling weak

* Cold skin

* Shivering

* Confusion

* Slow breathing

* Slow pulse

Treatment Your jobs are to:

* Summon help

* Reassure the casualty

* Gently rewarm her

Proceed as follows:

1 If you can get the casualty indoors, but if
this is not possible get her out of the wind.

2 Ask her permission to remove any wet or frozen clothing (cut it off if necessary).

3 Replace it with warm clothing – as many layers as possible.

4 If you are in an emergency situation and there is no warm clothing available, but someone has a 'space blanket', wrap the patient in this.

5 Cover the top of her head with something – a woolly hat is ideal.

6 If there is a bed available, get the casualty into it and cover her with layers of blankets, duvets, etc.

7 Do not offer a hot water bottle – these can be harmful in hypothermia.

8 If you have a thermometer, take the casualty's temperature as she recovers, and write down the result and the time.

9 If she is conscious, give her sips of warm drinks, provided she's not injured.

CONCUSSION
If a blow to the head interferes with the functioning of the brain, so that the casualty is knocked out or becomes confused, you must assume that he is concussed.

In all such cases the casualty MUST go to hospital, be seen by a doctor, and have a skull x-ray. Your main job is to make sure that this happens. Unfortunately, many people behave very foolishly where head injuries are concerned, and try to avoid going to hospital. In sport, some casualties even want to play on – this must be prevented.

If a person is knocked out and remains unconscious for more than a minute, then get someone to call an ambulance. Meanwhile, proceed as described in the section on **Unconsciousness**.

CONVULSIONS

Convulsions (fits) are most often the result of epilepsy (see **Epilepsy**), though in babies, a convulsion may simply be caused by a high temperature. (Babyhood convulsions are dealt with separately below.)

In a convulsion, the person loses consciousness, falls to the ground, and shakes all over. She may bite her tongue and possibly pass urine.

Your main job is to protect her until she is fully recovered. Proceed as follows:

1 Clear a space around the casualty, and discourage bystanders from crowding in.

2 Make her as comfortable as possible by putting cushions or rolled up coats under her head, and loosen the clothing around her neck (see Figure 1).

3 Do not let anybody try to put something between her teeth. This is a popular practice

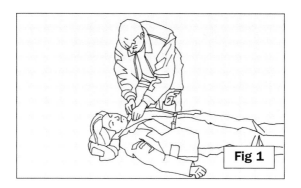

Fig 1

among uninformed people, but it is useless and dangerous.

4 When the casualty comes round, put her in the recovery position, as described in the section on **Unconsciousness.**

5 Stay with her until she is completely capable of looking after herself – or until skilled help arrives.

6 Most people who have epilepsy do not want to be taken to hospital in an ambulance – they just want to recover and get on with their daily lives. So only call an ambulance in the following circumstances:

> * If the person says she has never had a fit before
>
> * If she has another fit shortly after coming round
>
> * If the convulsion goes on for more than about 5 minutes

* If on recovery, she is obviously too confused to look after herself

Babyhood convulsions These usually occur because the child has a high temperature – babies' brains cannot cope with excessive heat. Proceed as follows:

1 Place the child somewhere comfortable, and protect her till she comes round.

2 As soon as possible, take her temperature and make a note of it.

3 Phone for a doctor, and tell him what the child's temperature is.

4 If her temperature is raised, make every effort to cool the child down, in the following ways:

* Turn off electric fires, etc

* Remove blankets and duvets

* Remove all clothing except pants

* Use an electric fan or a hairdryer on a cool setting to blow air on the child's body

You may find that relatives – particularly elderly ones – are outraged by these measures, and want to wrap the child up warmly 'so she doesn't get a chill'. Explain to them that doing this will raise her temperature and probably cause further fits.

5 Comfort and reassure the child until the doctor arrives.

CUTS AND GRAZES
If someone has a minor cut or graze, all you need do is wash the area carefully with soap and water, taking care to get rid of any dirt or grit in the wound. Then dry the skin gently, and cover the area with a sticking plaster (*see* **Sticking Plasters**).

Deep cuts should always been seen by a doctor. For cuts which are bleeding a lot, *see* **Bleeding**.

DISLOCATIONS
A dislocation occurs when a bone comes out of its socket. Common sites are the shoulders and fingers.

There is great pain, and you can usually see that the bone is out of place. Do not – repeat not – try to put the bone back into its socket. This is definitelt not a job for an untrained person.

What you should do is make sure that the injured part is supported until the casualty gets to hospital.

In the case of a finger dislocation, this is best done using a hand bandage (described in the section on **Bandages**), preferably with some soft padding under it, and a sling (*see* **Slings**).

In the case of a shoulder dislocation, simply put the patient's arm in a sling (*see* **Slings**) and take him to hospital.

DROWNING
Rapid action by you may save a person's life. Do not delay, because death can occur very rapidly.

Rescue from water Specialised techniques of rescue from water are taught by sub-aqua clubs and lifesaving organisations, and are outside the scope of this short book. I strongly recommend that you take a lifesaving course if one is available at your local swimming pool or beach.

Your basic aim should be to get the victim out of the water without drowning yourself in the process (sadly, it is not unusual for this to happen to rescuers).

If possible, get the person out while remaining on dry land yourself – for example, by throwing her a lifebelt on a rope. (Take care not to strike her with the lifebelt.)

If you have to go into the water:

> * Make every effort to calm the victim

> * Try to draw her to the shore from behind

> * If she stops breathing, try to give her mouth-to-mouth respiration in the water (*see* **Mouth-to-Mouth**)

As soon as the victim is out of the water, get her head lower than her body – this helps fluid to drain out – and make sure that an ambulance has been called.

Treatment Once the victim is ashore, proceed as follows:

1 Place her on a reasonably flat surface, with her head lower than the rest of her body.

2 Clear her mouth of anything that might cause a blockage, such as seaweed or dentures.

3 See if she is breathing. If she is, then keep her in the recovery position (described in the section on *Unconsciousness*) until medical help arrives, and ensure that she is wrapped up warmly. (See Figure 1.)

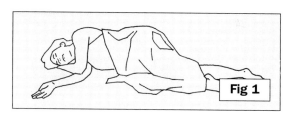

Fig 1

4 If she is not breathing, then you must:

* Check her airway, as described in the section on *Unconsciousness*

* Give her artificial respiration, as described in the section on *Mouth-to Mouth*.

5 If the casualty's heart has stopped, it is vital to give heart massage as well (*see* **Heart Massage**).

Note: Do not give up. People who appear to be dead have often been brought round by determined first aiders.

DRUG ABUSE
Sadly, substance abuse is all too common these days, so you may well encounter someone who is ill because they have taken too much of an illegal drug. Very often, a drug abuser is found unconscious – perhaps with pills or some other drug 'kit' beside him or in his bag or pockets. A person who injects drugs is very likely to have visible bruises and needle marks up his arms. Proceed as follows:

1 Get someone to call an ambulance.

2 Make sure the victim's airway is clear, as described under **Unconsciousness**.

3 If he has stopped breathing, give him artificial respiration (*see* **Mouth-to-Mouth**). If you are worried about being infected with hepatitis B or HIV virus you can use a protective shield or face mask.

4 If his heart has stopped, give cardiac massage (*see* **Heart Massage**).

5 If the victim is breathing, put him in the recovery position, as described in the section on **Unconsciousness**.

6 Collect any pills, drug 'gear', etc., for identification by doctors, taking great care not to jab yourself on any needles.

DRUNKENNESS

A conscious drunk can be dangerous to other people, so take care when you offer help to someone in this condition. Your main objectives are to calm her down, and to try to make sure that she doesn't harm herself, or others. Avoid arguing.

If possible, remove her car keys for safe keeping, and put any potential weapons out of reach. If necessary, call the police.

Drunks very frequently vomit, so be prepared for this to happen.

A person who is unconscious as a result of alcohol is in serious danger of dying – most commonly by choking on their own vomit. So proceed as follows:

1 Call for an ambulance.

2 Keep the patient's airway open, as described in detail in the section on *Unconsciousness*.

3 Be prepared to give cardiac massage (*see* *Heart Massage*) if the heart stops, and to give artificial respiration if breathing stops (*see* *Mouth-to-Mouth*).

4 Protect the casualty from the cold with blankets, etc.

5 Look out for other injuries – it is easy to overlook the fact that a drunken person has a wound on the head or elsewhere.

ELECTRIC SHOCK
The most important thing here is to make sure that neither you nor any other rescuer gets killed or hurt by the electricity.

Electric shock from power lines or overhead cables This kind of electricity 'jumps', so do not let anyone go within 20 metres of the victim until the electrical company has turned off the power. From then on, proceed as below.

Electric shock from home appliances If the casualty is still in contact with the electricity, DO NOT TOUCH HIM UNTIL YOU HAVE TURNED OFF THE POWER AT THE MAINS OR SWITCH. If this isn't possible, then use something wooden to push the victim away from the current, as in Figure 1. (Take great care not to stand on a wet floor as you do this.)

Then, when the casualty is safely away from the electricity, proceed as follows:

1 Call an ambulance.

2 If the casualty is unconscious, check his breathing and his pulse, and be prepared to give him both artificial respiration (*see Mouth-to-Mouth*) and cardiac massage (*see Heart Massage*).

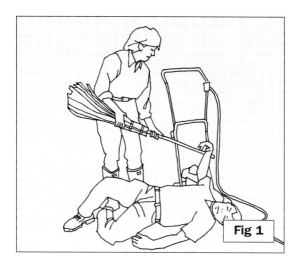

Fig 1

3 Once he is breathing normally, put him in the recovery position, as described in the section on *Unconsciousness*.

4 Stay with him until the ambulance arrives.

EPILEPSY

Epilepsy – which is extremely common – is a condition in which there are sudden electrical discharges in the brain. Very frequently, these cause convulsions (fits). The first aid procedure for these is described under the heading *Convulsions*.

There are other types of epilepsy in which the person does not have a fit. She may just suddenly look blank for a little while, and then 'come round' again. Or she may make repeated twitching movements.

In all such cases, what you need to do is stay with the person, and keep her calm and safe from injury until she has fully recovered. If in doubt, call medical help.

EYE INJURIES

Always regard an eye injury as potentially serious, because an eye wound can easily lead to permanent blindness.

If there is even the slightest doubt about whether an injury might be serious, you must ensure that the victim is taken to hospital as soon as possible.

In the meantime, keep him calm and ask him not to move his eyes around. If you have a 'pad-and-bandage' designed for eye use, apply it. Do not try to remove anything which is embedded in the eye.

FAINTING

A major problem with fainting is that well-meaning bystanders will often make vigorous attempts to do the wrong thing – which is to sit the victim up in a chair, or even stand her up.

Resist all such attempts. The correct treatment is to keep the faint victim lying down until she has fully recovered.

You can speed recovery by propping her legs up on something, as in Figure 1. Loosen clothing around the neck, and make sure she has plenty of air.

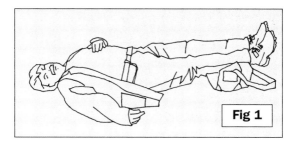

Fig 1

Note: Do also check for any injuries that may have been sustained during the fall.

FIRST AID KIT
It is a really good idea to keep a proper first aid kit in your car or kitchen (or both).

These days, you can buy fully equipped first aid outfits from pharmacies. But if you want to make your own, then the first essential is a really stout box, preferably with a carrying handle. The box should be brightly coloured – so that people can find it fast – and it should have the sort of catch that children cannot open.

Do not let other people help themselves from it casually, and if you have to use items from it yourself, make sure that you replace them promptly. There is nothing worse than finding that something vital is missing when you are dealing with an emergency.

A good plan is to write down all the contents of your first aid kit on a piece of paper. Stick this to the inside of the lid, so that anyone who opens it can see what's available.

Suggested items for a first aid kit
(see Figure 1)

* Stout box (see notes above)

* Torch (invaluable for giving first aid in the dark, e.g after a road accident)

* Batteries for torch (check regularly)

* Pen and paper – vital when sending messages about casualties

* Space blanket (for keeping the casualty warm)

* Ten safety pins (various sizes)

* Four crepe bandages

* Four small cotton bandages

* Two triangular bandages – mainly for slings (see **Slings**).

* Small box of sticking plasters (various sizes)

* Six sterile dressings (various sizes)

* Pack of cotton wool

* Pack of lint

* Pack of gauze pads

* One pad-and-bandage for eye injuries

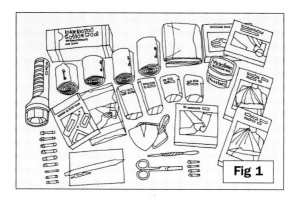

Fig 1

* Pack of wound-cleaning wipes

* Jar of Vaseline – extremely useful for all sorts of minor scrapes

* Small pair of sharp scissors (straight)

* Small tweezers

FISH HOOKS
Fish hooks cause particularly troublesome injuries to human beings, because their design makes them extremely difficult to remove from the wound.

Do not try to take out an embedded fish hook unless you are several hours from medical aid. Under normal circumstances, proceed as follows:

1 Put some clean padding (cotton wool or gauze) around the fish hook, so that it is held steady.

2 Bandage gently over the padded area.

3 Get the casualty to a doctor.

If there will not be any skilled medical help available for several hours, then proceed as follows:

1 If the barb is still under the skin (i.e. you cannot see it), try to draw the hook back along the line of entry – sometimes you can do this by looping some of the fishing line around the curve of the hook, and pulling on it gently.

2 If the barb has gone through the skin and come out again (i.e. if you can see it), then cut it off with a pair of wirecutters, as shown in Figure 1. It will then be easy to slide the rest of the hook out.

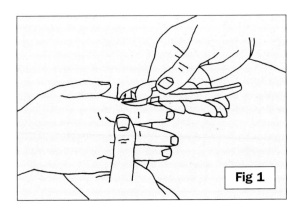

Fig 1

3 Clean and bandage the wound, and ensure that the casualty sees a doctor as soon as possible.

FITS (*see **Convulsions***)

FOREIGN BODIES
The term 'foreign body' means anything from
a nail to a marble – in other words, anything
that shouldn't be there.

Foreign bodies in the skin For fish hooks,
see the separate entry on ***Fish Hooks***.

Splinters If you can see the outer end of
the splinter, get a pair of clean tweezers and
withdraw it along the line of entry. If the
splinter is embedded deeper than that,
do not dig around – take the casualty to
a doctor.

Other foreign bodies in the skin Always get
medical advice.

Foreign bodies in the eye It is OK to
remove small pieces of grit, dust, etc., but
do not remove anything which is embedded.
The best way to get rid of specks of grit and
dust and small insects is to wash the eye
out with clean water (preferably with the chill
taken off it), using an eyebath.

Foreign bodies in the ear Many foreign bodies (e.g insects) can be successfully washed
out with clean, tepid water. If this doesn't
work, consult a doctor.

FRACTURES
These are exactly the same as breaks (*see
Broken Bones*).

FROSTBITE

In frostbite, there is very serious damage to body tissues, usually in the extremities.

Do not do any of the following, which are sometimes suggested as 'remedies':

* Do not put snow on the frostbitten part

* Do not rub it

* Do not put a hot water bottle or other strong source of heat on it

Instead, rewarm the affected part gently. This is best done by wrapping it in many layers of bandaging. In an emergency, you can put the frostbitten part under your own clothes, and against your skin. ALWAYS GET MEDICAL HELP. (*see **Cold (Extreme)***)

GAS POISONING

The type of household gas that is used in Britain and many other countries these days is not poisonous (although it is explosive), but poisoning by other types of gas – such as industrial gases and car exhaust gas – occur frequently. Your aim is to save the casualty's life, without losing your own. Proceed as follows:

1 Make sure that somebody has called for an ambulance.

2 Get the casualty out of the gas-filled environment (room, car, etc.): without breathing in the gas yourself. Alternatively, it may be possible to make the environment safe by rapidly opening all the doors and windows. DO NOT BREATHE IN UNTIL THIS HAS BEEN DONE.

3 Proceed as described in the section on *Unconsciousness*.

HEAD INJURY

Head injuries are much more dangerous than most people realise. Indeed any head injury can pose a threat to the victim's life, or to long-term health.

If the patient has been knocked out (even for a few seconds) or if he seems to be confused, then proceed as described in the section on *Concussion*.

Even if he has not been knocked out and is not confused, it is as well to keep a careful eye on him for the next 24 hours. Any sudden deterioration in his condition demands immediate medical attention.

HEART ATTACK

This is one of the most common illnesses in Western countries – and unfortunately a very frequent cause of death. It mainly occurs in people over 40, but occasionally occurs in younger people too.

The most common symptom is a severe, crushing pain in the centre of the chest, and the victim often collapses.

Accurate diagnosis of a heart attack takes years of training, but if you suspect one, proceed as follows:

1 Make the person comfortable, and reassure her.

2 Make sure that medical help has been called. If you are in a vehicle, e.g. a car or bus, go straight to hospital.

3 If the victim is conscious, give her one ordinary aspirin to chew. Although this sounds a trivial measure, it can help get rid of clots in the tubes which supply the heart with blood.

4 If she becomes unconscious, check that she has a pulse and is breathing, then proceed as described in the section on *Unconsciousness.*

HEART MASSAGE

Heart massage is used only when the casualty's heart has stopped beating. If the casualty has no pulse and no heartbeat, assume that the heart has stopped, and proceed as follows:

1 Get the victim lying flat on his back, on a firm surface (a bed will not usually do, because it will almost almost certainly be too soft).

2 Kneel beside him, and place the heel of your left hand on the lower end of his breastbone, as shown in Figure 1.

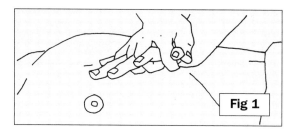

Fig 1

3 Put your right hand on top of the left one.

4 You must now drive your hands straight downwards about 5 cm (2 in), so that you compress the casualty's chest. Allow his chest to 'bounce' up again, but do not remove your hands. The technique is shown in Figure 2.

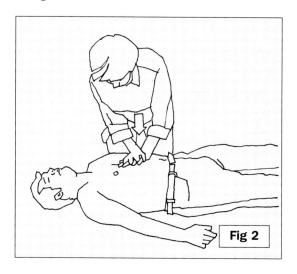

Fig 2

5 Repeat these compressions at a rate of slightly faster than one per second.

HEAT STROKE

Heat stroke is common in hot countries, but it can also occur in temperate lands, especially if people are working in enclosed, crowded spaces. A type of heat stroke occurs at 'ecstasy raves', where – thanks to the drug and the exertion of dancing in a packed room – a person's body temperature may rise to 41.7°C (107°F).

Symptoms include headache, confusion, very hot skin (without sweating) and, eventually, collapse. Your job is to get medical help, and to cool the victim down. Having called for a doctor or ambulance, proceed as follows:

1 Get the victim out of the heat and into a cool, shady place. If possible, take her temperature, and make a note of it.

2 Remove her clothes. If there is a fan or hairdryer available, blow cool air on her.

3 Put a sheet or other thin cloth over her trunk, and sprinkle it with cold water.

4 If the victim becomes unconscious, proceed as described in the section on *Unconsciousness*.

HYPOTHERMIA *(see Cold (Extreme))*

HYSTERIA

We are not dealing here with 'hysterical illnesses', i.e. illnesses that are real to the patient, but which have no physical basis.

We are talking about the kind of dramatic, out-of-control behaviour that people often show after a bereavement or a road accident, for example. They scream and shout and weep, and may do irrational things like tearing their clothes.

In these circumstances, keep calm yourself. Do not go in for the old Hollywood trick of slapping an hysterical person across the face. It is unlikely to do any good, it may cause an injury, and it will certainly make you liable to a charge of assault.

Instead, proceed as follows:

1 Talk calmly to the person.

2 Reassure him that everything will be OK.

3 If it seems appropriate, gently put an arm round him (do not physically restrain him unless there is a danger that he might harm himself – which is uncommon).

4 Keep talking until he calms down or medical help arrives.

(*see also* **Panic Attacks**)

JELLYFISH STINGS

These can be painful, and very occasionally they provoke a severe reaction and the victim collapses. Treat as follows:

1 Pour any type of alcohol (or vinegar) over the sting – but not near the eyes.

2 If you can get hold of some bicarbonate of soda (baking powder), mix it with water on a pad (e.g. a clean handkerchief), and apply it to the affected area.

3 If the sting is still causing pain, get the victim to a doctor or hospital.

4 If the victim becomes unconscious, proceed as described in the section on **Unconsciousness.**

KISS OF LIFE (see **Mouth-to-Mouth**)

MOUTH-TO-MOUTH
This type of artificial respiration has saved countless lives. Use it if a casualty has stopped breathing.

Note that if her heart has stopped beating as well, the casualty must be given cardiac massage (see **Heart Massage**) in addition to mouth-to-mouth.

This is easier if there are two of you – one to do heart massage and one to give mouth-to-mouth. Give one breath of mouth-to-mouth after every five thrusts of heart massage.

To give mouth-to-mouth to an adult or school-age child, proceed as follows:

1 Clear any obstruction from the casualty's mouth, as shown in Figure 1. Common obstructions include things like seaweed, false or broken teeth and vomit.

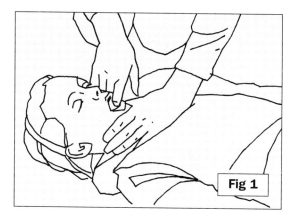

Fig 1

2 Ensure her airway is clear, as described in the section on **Unconsciousness**.

3 Adopt the position of the first aider shown in Figure 2. Note that he has closed off the casualty's nose between finger and thumb, and is supporting her chin with his other hand. To close of the caualty's nose, you need to squeeze the soft part just above the nostrils.

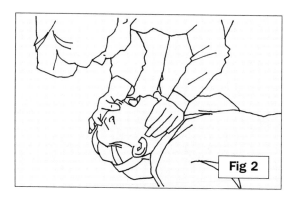

Fig 2

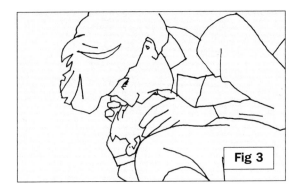

Fig 3

4 Now bend forwards and put your lips over the casualty's mouth, as in Figure 3. Blow into her mouth until you see her chest rise. Note that the first aider in the picture is keeping an eye on the chest, to see when it rises. It should only take a second.

5 Once the casualty's chest has risen, remove your mouth – and she should breathe out naturally.

6 Reapply your mouth and blow air in as before. Aim to give her one breath every 5 or 6 seconds.

7 Continue until the casualty starts breathing, or until medical help arrives.

Treating babies If you are saving a baby's (or toddler's) life, the technique is slightly different:

> * Instead of just putting your mouth over the casualty's mouth, put it over her nose and mouth.

* Give very gentle and small breaths –
  about as much air as you can hold in
  your puffed-out cheeks.

* Because babies need to breathe
  faster than adults, aim for one puff
  every 3 seconds.

NECK INJURY

Neck injuries can be very serious, because
there is often a risk of damage to the
spinal cord.

So if you think that a person may have had
a severe neck injury, DO NOT MOVE HIM.
Proceed as described in the section on
Back Injury. Make sure you do not let
enthusiastic helpers shift the casualty
around. Send them off to telephone for
medical help.

NOSEBLEED

Nosebleeds are common, and can be
frightening for the casualty – especially if it
is a young child. Proceed as follows:

1 Reassure the person that everything is
going to be all right, and that the bleeding
will stop.

2 Sit the victim up, with her head bent a
little forward.

3 Get her to breathe through her mouth –
not through her nose.

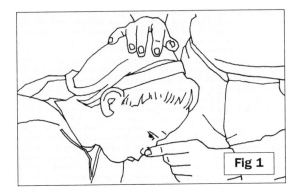

Fig 1

4 Use your forefinger and thumb to squeeze the soft part of the nose together firmly, as shown in Figure 1.

5 It is important to keep up this pressure for 15 minutes. Resist the temptation to let go for a second and have a peek.

6 At the end of this time, the bleeding should have stopped. If it hasn't, apply the pressure again, and then take the casualty to hospital .

A calm casualty can apply the pressure herself. The ancient remedy of putting a key down the casualty's back will be of no use.

After you have cured the nosebleed, advise the patient not to blow her nose for several hours.

OVERDOSE
Overdoses of drugs (prescribed or illegal) are common. Always take them seriously – never

assume that if you do nothing, the casualty will soon feel better and everything will be all right.

The conscious casualty If the person is conscious, your job is to get him to hospital. Take any unswallowed tablets, bottles, etc. with you – these will be a great help to the doctors. Do not attempt to make the casualty sick.

The unconscious casualty Call for an ambulance, then check the casualty's airway, as descibed in the section on *Unconsciousness.*

If necessary, give cardiac massage (*see* *Heart Massage*) and/or artificial respiration (*see* *Mouth-to-Mouth*).

If the casualty is breathing normally, and he has a pulse, place him in the recovery position, as described in the section on *Unconsciousness.*

Save any pills, medicines, etc. – and also anything which has been vomited up. (*see also* *Aspirin Overdose* and *Paracetamol Overdose*)

PANIC ATTACKS
Panic attacks are extremely common, and are nothing to be ashamed of.

The sufferer may be embarrassed, and could be reluctant to tell you if she has had such attacks in the past.

Symptoms include shaking, breathlessness, thumping in the chest, faintness, tingling and a feeling that something dreadful is happening. Many victims believe they are having a heart attack.

These symptoms are genuine, and are caused by changes in body chemistry. So do not waste time telling the person to 'snap out of it' or 'pull themselves together'. This may actually make them worse.

Proceed as follows:

1 Sit the sufferer down in a quiet place, away from onlookers.

2 Talk to her calmly, and reassure her that you will look after her, and that everything will be all right.

3 Ask if she has had previous attacks. If she has, then gently point out that she survived those, and will survive this one.

4 If she is breathing fast, suggest that it would be a good idea to breathe in and out from a paper bag for 20 seconds or so. (Do not use a plastic bag).

5 When she has calmed down, encourage her to see a doctor that day.

PARACETAMOL OVERDOSE
It is alarmingly easy to overdose with paracetamol (Panadol), so always stick to the stated dose. Be wary of the fact that

many proprietary remedies contain paracetamol among their ingredients.

One of the biggest dangers with this drug is the fact that a person who has taken an overdose may seem perfectly well for some days – but then collapse and die.

So anyone who has swallowed an overdose of paracetamol MUST be taken to hospital as soon as possible.

Symptoms In the early stages following an overdose, there may be no symptoms at all, though many people experience nausea and vomiting. There may also be pain in the upper part of the abdomen (tummy). The patient usually then remains well until collapsing with liver problems.

Treatment If the person is conscious, get him to hospital right away, taking any unused tablets or empty tablet bottles with you.

Do not try to make him vomit, but if vomiting does occur, try and take a 'sample' with you for analysis.

If the person is unconscious, turn to the section on *Unconsciousness* and proceed as described there. Do not let anyone destroy any suicide notes, unused tablets or empty bottles.

RECOVERY POSITION (see under *Unconsciousness*)

SEXUAL ASSAULT

Sexual assault is deeply distressing for the victim. So one of the most important things you can do is reassure her, and let her know that you will look after her and that help has been summoned.

If the victim is female and you are male, it may well be that your presence makes her feel threatened – so you should try and find a female 'chaperone'.

A major difference between sexual assault and other forms of injury is this: **it is vital not to remove any forensic evidence**.

Therefore, do not wipe away bloodstains, or start cleaning up around cuts and scratches. Try to persuade the victim not to wash herself (including her hands) until after expert help has arrived.

Remember that a phone call to the local Rape Crisis Centre may be invaluable, since it should be staffed by people who are experienced in counselling and comforting victims of sexual assault.

SHOCK

The word 'shock' has two meanings: *emotional* shock and *physical* shock.

Emotional shock After a dramatic event (such as a sudden bereavement), many people are mentally stunned and a little confused. The best treatment is to calm them and reassure them.

Do not try and get them to swallow alcohol, which may just make things worse.

If you are certain that they are not injured, a cup of tea is often soothing and warming.

Physical shock This is quite different; it is a medical condition which often happens after a severe injury, bleeding or a heart attack. It is very serious, and if you respond quickly, you may save a life.

The symptoms are:

* Faintness

* Paleness (often greyness in fair-skinned people)

* Cold and clammy skin

* Collapse

* Fast, shallow breathing

* Fast but 'thready' pulse

Treatment Resist anyone who has old-fashioned ideas about giving the casualty hot, sweet tea, or alcohol.

Proceed as follows:

1 Make sure that somebody has called for an ambulance.

2 Treat any obvious cause of shock – such as severe bleeding (*see* **Bleeding**).

3 Get the casualty lying face up (Figure 1), with his legs propped up a couple of feet or so (around 60 cm) above the level of his head. This encourages blood to drain back from the legs towards the heart.

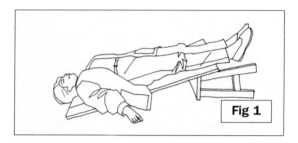

Fig 1

4 Loosen tight clothing. Protect the casualty from the cold. If he becomes unconscious, proceed as described in **Unconsciousness.**

SLINGS, AND ELEVATED SLINGS
These are very useful for supporting an injured arm or hand. Use a triangular bandage, found in a standard first aid kit, or make one by folding any large square of cloth diagonally - a women's square scarf is ideal. In the instructions that follow, it is assumed you have a triangular cloth

Ordinary slings These are useful for arm or wrist injuries They can also be used in cases of dislocated shoulder (*see* **Dislocations**). Proceed as follows:

1 Make sure the casualty's arm is supported, and then place the triangle behind her forearm, as shown in Figure 1.

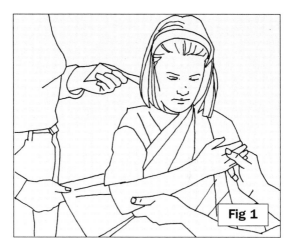

Fig 1

2 Bring the lowest corner of the triangle up (Figure 2) – and tie it to the topmost point of the triangle behind the casualty's neck.

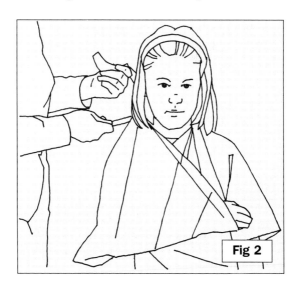

Fig 2

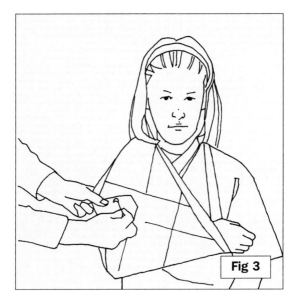

Fig 3

3 Pin the remaining corner of the triangle in front of the elbow with a safety-pin (Figure 3).

Elevated slings These are good for hand or shoulder injuries. Proceed as follows:

1 Make sure that you (or a helper) are supporting the injured arm

2 If there is nobody else to assist you, it is often possible to get the casualty to support the injured arm with her other hand.

3 Ask the casualty to put her hand on the opposite shoulder, as in Figure 4.

4 Spread the triangular bandage over the front of the arm, as shown in Figure 5.

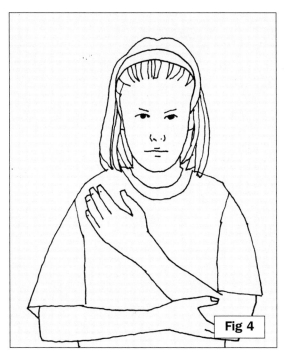

Fig 4

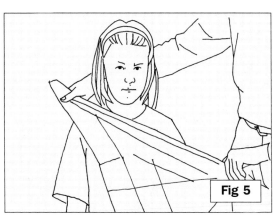

Fig 5

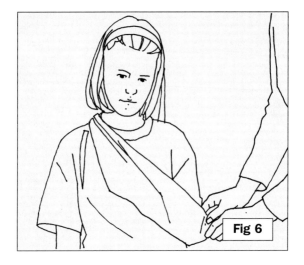

Fig 6

4 Carefully supporting the casualty's elbow, tuck the lower edge of the triangle behind it, as in Figure 6.

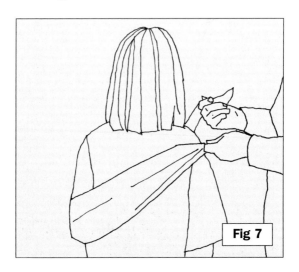

Fig 7

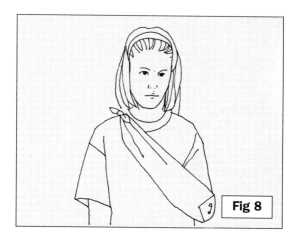

Fig 8

5 Take the lowest part of the triangular bandage up around the casualty's back, and tie the points together, as shown in Figure 7.

6 Tuck the remaining point in at the elbow, and fix it with a safety-pin. The final appearance is shown in Figure 8.

SMOKE INHALATION
Smoke inhalation (e.g. from a house fire) can kill someone very quickly. Indeed, most 'fire deaths' are actually caused by smoke. Proceed as follows:

1 Make sure someone has called the emergency services.

2 Get the casualty out of the smoke and into fresh air (however, make sure that you yourself are not overcome by smoke in the process).

3 If the casualty is unconscious or becomes unconscious, proceed as described in the section on **Unconsciousness.**

4 Treat burns (*see* **Burns**).

SNAKE BITE
Most snake bites – particularly in temperate countries – are not as serious as people fear. However, they can cause death, so always treat them with caution.

Do not try any 'film tricks', such as cutting into the wound with a knife and trying to suck the venom out. This will only make things worse. Instead, proceed as follows:

1 Lie the victim down. If you can do this in a large estate car that can be used to transfer him to hospital, so much the better.

2 Keep the casualty calm.

3 If water (better still, soapy water) is available, wash the wound.

4 Remove anything which could be constricting the bitten part. For example, if the bite is on the hand, remove watches bangles and rings. This is because the bitten part may soon swell up.

5 Support the injured part with your hands, or with a sling (*see* **Slings**), until you get to medical help.

Note: In some countries, notably France, supplies of life-saving 'anti-venom' injections are kept at chemists' shops in areas where there are snakes.

SPIKY FISH

Even in temperate waters, it is common for paddlers to step on spiky fish (weaver fish), which lie hidden in the sand. The resulting puncture wounds in the sole of the foot are very painful.

Put the injured foot in hot water – as hot as the casualty can stand – for half an hour. This helps to neutralise the fish venom.

As soon as practicable, get the casualty to a hospital or doctor, so that any spines in her foot can be removed.

STICKING PLASTER

There should be a variety of these in any first aid kit (*see First Aid Kit*).

Before applying one, ask the casualty if he is allergic to sticking plaster – many people are. If so, it is best to use a 'hypo-allergenic' plaster or, failing that, a small bandage.

Waterproof sticking plasters must be used in certain circumstances – for example, when the casualty is swimming, or if he is a food-handler.

To apply a sticking plaster, remove any outer wrapping. Then start to peel back the two protective strips, without touching the pad.

Put the pad on the skin (which should be dry). It is usually best to apply the plaster at right angles to the cut, because this helps to draw the edges of the wound together.
Pull off the two protective strips, and then press down on the non-padded parts of the plaster, especially round the edges.

STINGS
Please note that this section does not deal with bites from snakes (which are not stings); they covered in the section on *Snake Bites*.

For stings from fish spikes,(*see **Spiky Fish***).

There are three common types of sting which you may encounter: nettle stings; bee stings; and wasp stings.

Nettle stings These are distressing to children (and not much fun for adults), but their effect does not usually last for very. However, if you are really badly stung, you may experience unpleasant tingling for some days afterwards.

The best treatment is to put on something cooling, such as a flannel soaked in cold water. Calamine lotion is soothing. Many people swear by dock leaves, though it is doubtful if they do anything more than provide coolness.

Do not apply ointments or creams containing medication; they will not do any good, and may even provoke a sensitivity reaction.

Bee stings The sting will usually be in the skin. Remove it gently with tweezers. Do not squeeze the top part of it, as this will inject more venom into the victim.

Then apply a pad soaked in cold water. If the victim is in intense pain, aspirin (not for children) or paracetamol will help to relieve it

There are pain-relieving treatments available, mostly sprays that contain local anaesthetic, but I do not recommend that you use them, because they can sometimes cause very distressing skin reactions.

If the victim collapses after being stung by a bee, get someone to call an ambulance. Reassure her. If she becomes unconscious, proceed as described in the section on *Unconsciousness*.

Wasp stings Wasps do not leave a sting in the skin, so do not waste time trying to remove one. Apply a pad soaked in cold water, and if necessary give aspirin (not for children) or paracetamol. If the victim collapses, refer to the previous paragraph.

Local anaesthetic sprays for relieving the pain of wasp stings are widely sold; again they can cause a bad sensitivity reaction.

STROKES
Unfortunately, strokes are extremely common – especially in old people. Symptoms vary, but often the person suddenly becomes confused or may be

unable to speak. Some victims lose consciousness; many lose the ability to move one side of the body. Very frequently, the face is pulled to one side.

Your job is to call medical help, and to make sure that the casualty can breathe until that help arrives. Proceed as follows:

1 If the person is conscious, just lie him flat, keep him comfortable, and try to reassure him.

2 If the casualty is unconscious, proceed as described in the section on *Unconsciousness*.

UNCONSCIOUSNESS

If somebody is unconscious, then the situation is potentially serious, because there is always a chance that an unconscious person will die, especially if she is left alone. **Therefore, it is vital not to leave an unconscious person alone.**

What can you do for an unconscious casualty? It is all summed up in the flow chart on the next page.

Now, let's go through the flow chart, item by item.

Is the casualty breathing? You can rapidly establish whether or not the casualty is breathing by listening close to her nose and mouth. It may also be helpful to put your fingertips near the nose and mouth.

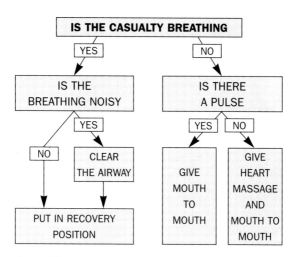

An old-fashioned way to check for breathing is to hold a mirror over the casualty's face to see if it mists up. However, this takes so long that the casualty might be dying by the time you have found out if she is breathing.

If in doubt, assume that she is not breathing, then move on to check for a pulse (see below).

Is the breathing noisy? If her breathing isn't noisy, then you can assume that her airway is not obstructed by anything. Just put her in the recovery position (see below).

But if the breathing is noisy – with grunts or a snoring noise – then you must act fast, because the noise means that the airway is obstructed by something.

The obstruction could be anything from broken teeth to a blood clot. Quite often, it is vomited material. Most frequently of all, it is the casualty's own tongue. Odd though that may sound, the human tongue can easily 'fall back', and choke an unconscious person, with fatal results.

The next section explains how to clear the casualty's airway.

Clearing the airway To clear the airway, the first thing you must do is use your finger to get rid of anything which is causing an obstruction in the mouth. Dentures can be left alone, provided that they haven't slipped out of place.

Next, you have to make sure that the tongue is not blocking the throat. In most people, it will block the throat if the head is in the position shown in Figure 1.

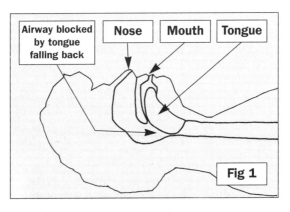

However, if the head is tilted back – as shown in Figure 2 – the tongue should not obstruct the airway.

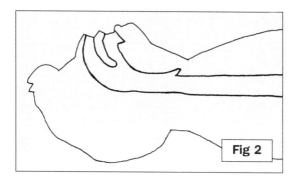

Fig 2

So, get the casualty's head well back and, as shown in Figure 3, keep it in position by putting one or two fingers under her chin. You have to tug quite hard in the direction shown by the arrow in order to make certain that the airway is clear. Do not ease up on this pressure: maintain it continuously until you are sure that the patient can breathe without any noise. Then you can put her in the recovery position (see below).

The recovery position Once the casualty is breathing normally and without noise, you can safely put her in the 'recovery position'.

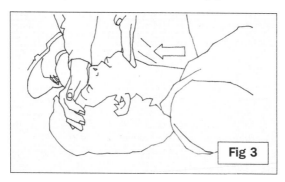

Fig 3

Note: Do not attempt to move her into the recovery position if there is a suspicion of a neck or spine injury).

One great advantage of the recovery position is that although you should still stay with the casualty, you will at least now be able to do other things, such as make calls on a mobile phone, or treat her other injuries.
Proceed as follows:

1 Let us assume that the casualty is lying on her back, as in Figure 1. Make sure you have checked that her airway is clear, as above. Then take hold of the arm nearest to you, and put it in a position where it looks as though she is giving a 'Halt' signal to traffic.

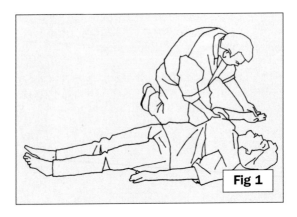

Fig 1

2 Reach over and get hold of the other arm by the elbow. Bring it up so that the back of her hand is against her cheek, as shown in Figure 2.

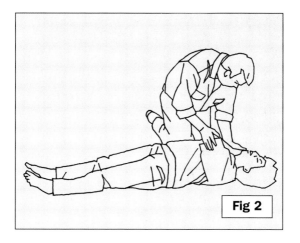

Fig 2

3 Use one of your hands to keep her arms in place, as shown in Figure 3. With your other hand, grasp her far leg, and pull it towards you. You will find this easiest if you grip it by the knee. If the casualty is heavy get someone to help.

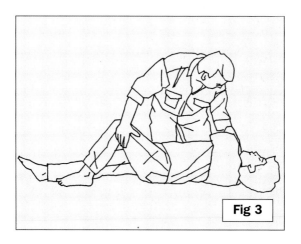

Fig 3

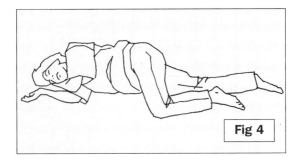

Fig 4

4 You should now find that she is lying in the comfortable position shown in Figure 4. This is the recovery position. Stay with her until help arrives.

Checking for a pulse Looking at the flow chart on page 87, you will see that if the unconscious casualty does not appear to be breathing, your next move must be to check for a pulse.

Even doctors find this difficult sometimes – particularly if the casualty is very overweight. The best rule is this: if you cannot detect any pulse after about 20 seconds, then it is best to assume that the heart has stopped, and to go ahead and give heart massage (see below).

To find a pulse, proceed as follows:

1 Always use the middle finger of your dominant hand, as this is the one most likely to detect a pulse accurately. Do not use your index finger; this already has your own pulse in it, which may confuse things.

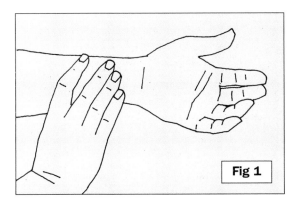

Fig 1

2 Begin by feeling on the inside of the casualty's wrist, as shown in Figure 1. If you have not found a pulse within 10 seconds, move on to step 3.

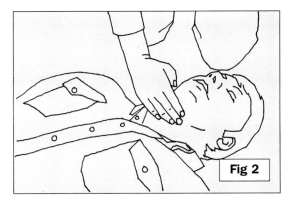

Fig 2

3 Feel for the pulse in the front of the casualty's neck, just to one side of the Adam's apple, as shown in Figure 2. If you cannot find a pulse within 10 seconds, move on to step 4.

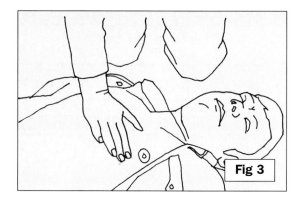

Fig 3

4 Before you actually start heart massage, it is worth spending a few seconds with the palm of your hand flat on the skin over the casualty's heart, as in Figure 3, in case you detect a heartbeat that way.

Mouth-to-mouth Proceed as described in the section on *Mouth-to-Mouth*.

Heart massage Proceed as described in the section on *Heart Massage*.

VAGINAL BLEEDING
Heavy vaginal bleeding can be distressing for a woman – and embarrassing for her as well. Unfortunately, some people are still not very understanding about this subject, so your main objectives are to:

> * Reassure the woman, and tell her that you will look after her

> * Make her comfortable

* Get medical help if you think that it is
necessary

Proceed as follows:

1 Get her to somewhere with some privacy,
away from bystanders.

2 Lie her down in a comfortable place,
raising her legs on a pile of pillows, cushions
or coats.

3 Get her some sanitary pads – a female
nearby may have some, but they are also
easily obtainable from chemists,
supermarkets, etc.

4 If there is a lot of bleeding, get somebody
to call for an ambulance.

VOMITING
If somebody starts to vomit, then proceed
as follows:

1 Give them a bowl or plastic bag.

2 Try to reassure them.

3 Between bouts of retching, make sure
that they are sitting or lying down in a
comfortable place.

4 If vomiting is repeated, or accompanied
by diarrhoea, always get medical advice.

Important If a person vomits up *black
material* or *blood*, this indicates a serious

problem in the region of the stomach. Get
the casualty to hospital, taking a sample
of the vomited material with you for the
doctors to inspect.